THE ILLUSTRATED
CORONARY FACT BOOK

The
ILLUSTRATED
CORONARY
FACT BOOK

by
Jesse E. Edwards, M.D.
Bernard Goott, M.D.

Edited by James R. Ullyot

Illustrated by Robert Benassi

AN ARCO BOOK

ARCO PUBLISHING COMPANY, INC.

219 Park Avenue South, New York, N.Y. 10003

An ARC Book
Published by Arco Publishing Company, Inc.
219 Park Avenue South, New York, N.Y. 10003

Library of Congress Catalog Card Number   72-96056

ISBN 0–668–02935–8

Printed in the United States of America

CONTENTS

Foreword

This little book presents in the shortest possible scope a clear picture of the main health problem that we face in the U.S.A. today, namely the disease of the large and medium-size arteries of the body, which we call atherosclerosis. This is a process of the gradual but usually steady and relentless accumulation of blood clots and fat superimposed on spots of wear and tear in the inside artery walls, finally narrowing the channels through which the blood flows to the extent that the heart muscle suffers from involvement of the coronary arteries and the brain suffers because of the involvement of the cerebral arteries. Heart attacks and strokes result, and in this day and age are affecting younger and younger adults.

We do not have all the answers but we know enough, as explained in this book, to begin to do something about it and not just lament our fate. We have done harder things than this, and there is no reason why we can't succeed. But we have got to roll up our sleeves and work at it.

Nature gave us muscles to use, and we have largely quit using them a million years too soon. Nature also gave us a brain, but we seem to be morons in applying just common sense to the problem. Let's get going!

Paul Dudley White, M.D.
Boston, Massachusetts

THE ILLUSTRATED
CORONARY FACT BOOK

Introduction

This book is about coronary heart disease, the major medical problem in the Western world today. Coronary heart disease is the general term which refers to coronary artery disease and its various possible effects: heart attack, angina, and related complications. So common is coronary artery disease, the underlying cause of heart attack and angina, that it has been called the twentieth-century epidemic.

Today's journalistic attention to heart attack persistently reminds us of the seriousness of this epidemic, as do the incidents among family and friends. Various articles on diet and theories as to the causes of coronary artery disease offer numerous suggestions for the prevention of coronary heart problems. Individuals affected by coronary heart disease often receive an assortment of advice from many sources on the matter of recovery.

Despite the availability of such information and suggestions, many people continue to show need for a more integrated and total understanding of coronary heart disease. Questions such as "What is a heart attack?" reflect their desire to learn more about the mechanics of coronary heart problems. They are also curious about the variety of conditions other than heart attack which may accompany

1

coronary artery disease. (One such condition, incidentally, is the absence of symptoms or illness.)

Many people are understandably confused by the vocabulary of coronary heart disease, which includes such terms as "acute myocardial infarction." Others who are concerned about recovery or prevention are not sure which items of information apply to their own lives.

This book is for all of these people, the intellectually curious as well as the emotionally concerned. The authors present an authoritative and concise review of the mechanics, terms, and various ramifications of coronary artery disease. The highly illustrated, easy-to-read presentation also brings to light facts which have proved helpful to countless individuals in the important areas of recovery and prevention. At the end, the authors take a look into the future.

The information in this book is designed as background to supplement, not replace, the specific advice of one's own physician. He alone knows the particular details which ultimately make each person's case unique.

The authors believe that a better informed public can assist the medical profession in restraining coronary heart disease. They emphasize, too, that while coronary artery disease may be of the most serious proportions to some, many with this problem can, with appropriate care, lead productive and happy lives.

1

The Normal Circulatory System

The heart is both the driving force of the normal circulatory system and an organ served by it.

Because the heart is so important in the circulation of blood, and because circulating blood is so important to the health of the heart, an understanding of the heart would be incomplete without an understanding of the circulatory system. To know the heart in terms of the circulatory system also allows an appreciation for the potentially far-reaching effects of heart abnormalities and for the basic circulatory nature of coronary artery disease.

The heart with its connected system of arteries and veins running throughout the body constitutes the vascular, or circulatory, system. The circulation of blood may be likened to a busy trucking service that picks up and delivers items along the same route on a repeating, nonstop basis (see Figure 1–1).

PICKUPS AND DELIVERIES

Among the pickup stations (see Figure 1–2) are the lungs, where the blood takes in all-important oxygen, and the intestinal tract and liver, where the blood picks up nourishment from food eaten.

After it has obtained nourishment, oxygen, and other essential materials, the blood delivers them to all parts of

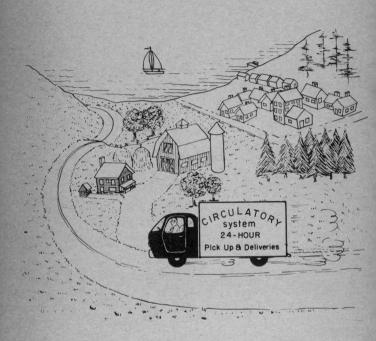

Figure 1-1.

the body, including the heart muscle, the brain, the muscles, and all the organs. Along its route the circulating blood also picks up certain waste materials and delivers them to the kidneys and liver. These last two organs direct the waste materials out of the body.

The pickups and deliveries repeat themselves as the blood circulates over and over again throughout the body.

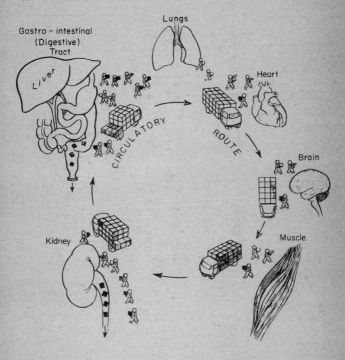

Figure 1-2.

Every organ in the body needs those continuous pickups and deliveries of circulating blood in order to survive and to perform its function. The heart is no exception.

The heart's job of keeping the circulating blood in motion makes it unique and absolutely essential.

2

The Normal Heart

TWO PUMPS

In a real pickup and delivery truck, the engine provides the force that moves the truck. In the body, two pumps provide the thrust which keeps the blood moving continuously. One is the *main pump* (the *left ventricle*). The other is an *auxiliary pump* (the *right ventricle*).

The main pump collects the blood from the lungs and sends it through the body. The auxiliary pump receives the blood from the body and sends it through the lungs.

Figure 2–1 shows the two pumps as separate hand pumps outside the body. Actually, they are parts of one organ, the heart.

The somewhat complicated real-life arrangement of the main and auxiliary pumps (left ventricle and right ventricle, respectively) appears in Figure 2–2, a view of the internal structure of the heart in its normal position. You are facing the heart as you would face another person. That person's left is to your right and vice versa. In other illustrations of the heart which follow, the same perspective applies.

Note that a wall separates the two pumps, also that each pump, or ventricle, is associated with a chamber (*atrium*) above it where blood accumulates before being received and expelled by the pump.

Knowledge of the interior structure of the heart and of the movement of blood through the main and auxiliary

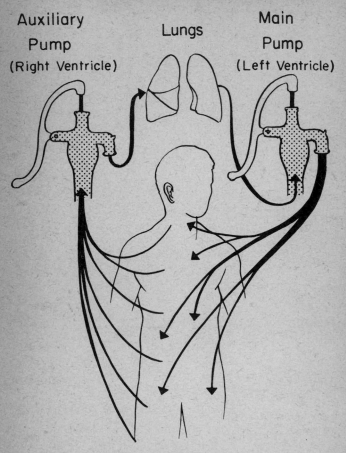

Auxiliary
Pump
(Right Ventricle)

Lungs

Main
Pump
(Left Ventricle)

Figure 2-1.

pumps helps in understanding how the heart performs its
key function of keeping the circulating blood in motion.
The shading and arrows in Figure 2–2 help to show the
movement of blood.

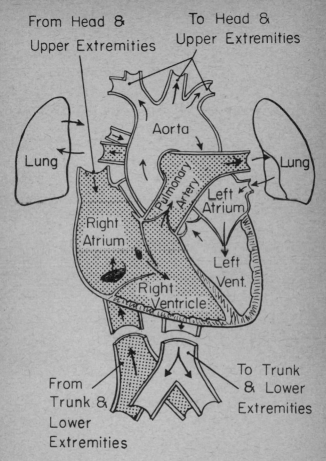

From Head &
Upper Extremities

To Head &
Upper Extremities

Aorta

Lung

Lung

Pulmonary Artery

Left
Atrium

Right
Atrium

Left
Vent.

Right
Ventricle

From
Trunk &
Lower
Extremities

To Trunk
& Lower
Extremities

Figure 2-2.

From the body, the *right atrium* receives deoxygenated, or "blue," blood (shaded in the drawing), which has given up oxygen to the tissues. This blood passes into the *right ventricle* (the auxiliary pump), which pumps it on to the lungs through a large vessel, the *pulmonary artery*. In the lungs, the blood accepts oxygen in a process called oxygenation.

After it has been oxygenated by the lungs, the oxygen-rich, or "red," blood returns to the *left atrium*, which delivers it to the *left ventricle* (main pump). The main pump then forces the blood to the entire body by way of a vessel called the *aorta* and its many branches.

The quality of the circulating blood depends on the competence of the lungs, a fact that turns attention to the important relationship between the heart and lungs in the circulatory system.

THE ROLE OF THE LUNGS

The oxygenation of blood is as vital as the delivery of blood to all parts of the body.

A delivery system without something to deliver is useless. And so the heart and lungs cooperate in a necessary partnership. Without properly functioning lungs to oxygenate the blood, the activity of a normal heart would be to no avail, for it would be pumping oxygen-deficient blood throughout the body.

In Figure 2–3, the heart is shown in the same position as in Figure 2–2. The lungs are shown so as to emphasize the connections with the heart. Once again, arrows indicate the direction of the flow of blood and shading helps to differentiate the sides of the heart.

The left side of the heart (unshaded) contains the main pump, which collects the freshly oxygenated blood from the lungs and sends it to the body. The right side (shaded) houses the auxiliary pump which collects deoxygenated blood from the body and sends it to the lungs.

In the lungs, the blood is resupplied with oxygen, which the body must have continuously in order for life to exist.

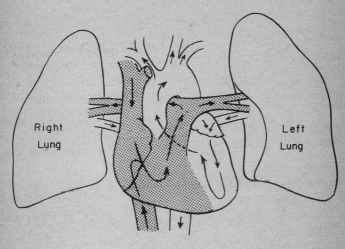

Figure 2-3.

THE IMPORTANCE OF COORDINATED CONTRACTIONS

The ventricles of the heart must pump effectively and unfalteringly. Each pump consists of millions of microscopic *muscle fibers*. Contraction of each of these fibers goes into the total pumping action. But the force of each contracting fiber by itself is infinitesimal. Therefore, coordinated contraction of the many muscle fibers is the key to the normal pumping action of the ventricles.

Lack of coordination gives an inefficient result as in the unsuccessful lift by the men depicted in Figure 2–4. But note what happens when the men work together in response to a signal caller (Figure 2–5).

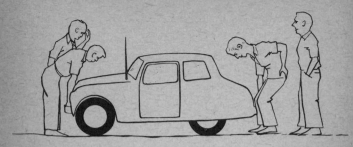

Figure 2-4.

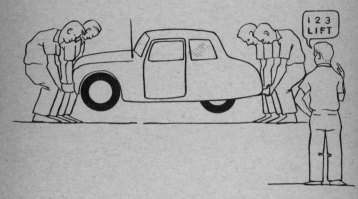

Figure 2-5.

There is a special *electrical signal system* in the heart which makes it work efficiently by stimulating the muscle fibers to contract in a coordinated and unified manner. This system is analogous to the signal caller in Figure 2–5. It determines the timing as well as the coordination of the contractions. You can recognize its effects by the regular intervals between your own pulse beats.

Any deviation from this regularity is called an *arrhythmia*. Some deviations from regularity of the pulse are not of major concern. Others are, especially when they accompany seriously uncoordinated contractions of the many individual heart fibers. At worst, a sudden breakdown of the signal system causes the heart muscle fibers to contract individually and at random so that the pumps merely quiver in an ineffective condition called *ventricular fibrillation*.

In a healthy heart, the coordinated contractions produce impressively strong performance. The normal left ventricle in an adult at rest pumps about 5 quarts of blood each minute or 1,300 gallons each day, and even more during exercise or work.

In addition to the properly functioning electrical system, the heart, if it is to be a strong and efficient pump, must have nutrition and oxygen supplied to its muscle fibers. The *coronary arteries* are the normal means by which the heart muscle receives its own nutrition and oxygen.

3

The Normal Coronary Arteries

Strong and reliable contractions of the ventricles depend upon healthy muscle fibers which make up the walls of the heart as well as a properly functioning signal system. The continuous supply of freshly oxygenated blood is needed by the heart muscle if it is to remain healthy and carry out its function.

As with other parts of the body, the blood supply to the heart muscle comes by way of arteries which branch from the *aorta*—not, as one might think, from directly inside the heart. The arteries serving the heart muscle are the *coronary arteries*.

In the last sense, the heart is like a gasoline tank truck which does not run on the gasoline it hauls. The truck must stop at service stations to get its own fuel (Figure 3–1).

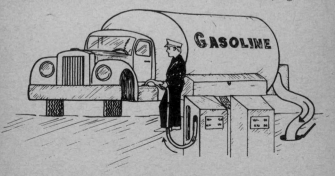

Figure 3-1.

Similarly, the heart contains large volumes of blood. But this blood cannot nourish the heart muscle until it leaves the heart and returns by way of the coronary arteries. In terms of the drawing, the line carrying gasoline into the underground storage tank may be likened to the aorta while the line carrying gasoline to the truck (heart) is a coronary artery.

There are two coronary arteries.° Each originates from the aorta. Their branches, which extend over the heart, penetrate and carry blood into the muscular wall of the heart as shown in Figure 3–2. Incidentally, the name "coronary" comes from the crown-like distribution of the arteries over the heart.

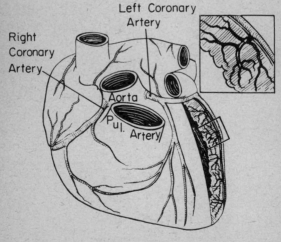

Figure 3-2.

°Physicians sometimes refer to three coronary arteries, the right coronary and the two main branches of the left coronary.

The two arteries are called right and left coronary arteries. Both serve the main pump, or left ventricle, principally. The left coronary artery primarily serves the front and sides of the left ventricle. The right coronary primarily serves the back of the left ventricle and the right ventricle. In Figure 3–2, the right coronary artery passes out of view on its way to the back of the heart and left ventricle.

In Figure 3–3, a portion of coronary artery is shown at its point of origin. In this location, the coronaries are usually about one-half the diameter of an ordinary lead pencil. Their branches are correspondingly smaller.

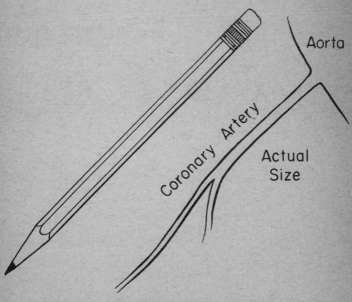

Figure 3-3.

Through the normal coronary artery, blood flows into the heart muscle to deliver oxygen and other nourishing substances. The flow is made possible in part by the great width of the bore relative to the diameter of the vessel, as shown in the magnified view of Figure 3–4. Another factor is an elasticity in the normal coronary artery which allows resilience in accommodating varying rates of blood flow and pressure.

These, then, are the normal coronary arteries: the lifelines providing the only route for delivery of oxygen and nourishment to heart muscle. When they are affected by disease, the flow of blood may become so negligible as to jeopardize the health and performance of heart muscle in serious and familiar ways (as in heart attack). It is the impairment of blood flow through the coronary arteries which is the underlying cause of all types of coronary heart disease.

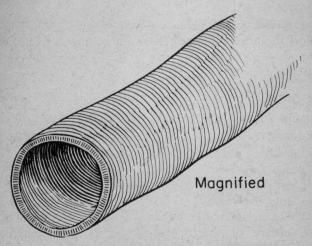

Magnified

Figure 3-4.

4

Coronary Artery Disease

Coronary artery disease, the fundamental basis for heart attack, is the development of areas of narrowing in the coronary arteries.

The narrowing may obstruct the flow of blood to such an extent that heart muscle suffers from lack of enough blood for proper function. Frequently called *hardening of the coronary arteries*, coronary artery disease carries the technical names *coronary arteriosclerosis* or *coronary atherosclerosis*.

Arteriosclerosis is characterized by areas of thickening along the artery's lining. These thickenings are caused by abnormal deposits of various substances, including fatty materials and fibrous tissue. Such deposits have been likened to rust accumulating along the lining in water pipes. Progressive accumulation of the deposits is associated with a corresponding reduction or narrowing of the bore (lumen) of the coronary artery, as shown in the two views of a diseased portion (Figure 4–1). Build-up of the abnormal deposits is also associated with a loss of the normal elasticity and with deposits of calcium in the artery, accounting for the term "hardening."

There are times when a *clot* (*thrombus*) may develop on the surface of the thickened portion and completely obstruct the channel, as shown in Figure 4–2.

19

Arteriosclerosis

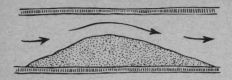

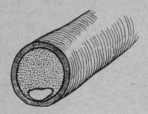

Figure 4-1.

Arteriosclerosis and Clot

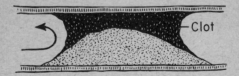

Clot

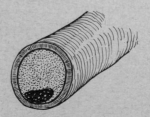

Figure 4-2.

HEART ATTACKS WITHOUT CLOTS

In the past, it was popularly believed that a clot had to develop in a coronary artery for a heart attack to occur. (The formation of such a clot is called a *coronary thrombosis.*) Recent research has shown, however, that in the presence of coronary arteriosclerosis, a heart attack can occur even without a clot.

In a heart attack, the heart muscle becomes damaged because of an inadequate supply of blood. A narrowed artery may allow some blood to reach the heart muscle, and such a supply may be adequate most of the time. But there are times of increased need when the narrowed channel may fail to allow enough blood through to meet the needs of heart muscle. The inadequate supply of blood at these times may combine with other factors to precipitate a heart attack. One example of a critical development would be a drop in blood pressure which could be caused, for example, by a bleeding ulcer. With less force behind it, the blood may slow down as it moves through the unyielding diseased coronary artery. Another example would be the individual's greater expenditure of energy, as in hard work. At such times the heart beats faster. The need for the delivery of oxygen and nourishment to heart muscle increases. But the narrowed coronary artery may not allow enough blood to flow through it and the heart muscle may suffer.

Several factors distinguish hardening of the coronary arteries from other diseases. Although the disease may cause a sudden crisis such as a heart attack, it develops gradually at varying rates of speed in each affected individual. The extent or rate of its development is extremely difficult, if not impossible, to diagnose at any time. Arteriosclerosis may be minimized in its development, but there is no practical or effective way to eliminate all of the various abnormal deposits in the arteries once they have appeared.

It would be quite reasonable to surmise that the majority of adult Americans have some deposits of the type which characterize hardening of the coronary arteries. But countless millions of people with varying degrees of arteriosclerosis have never experienced any heart problems. This underscores the fact that the presence of coronary arteriosclerosis does not mean a heart attack will occur. The chances of an attack are always present when coronary arteriosclerosis is known or suspected to exist. But when and in what form an attack will occur is impossible to predict because there are no clearly predictable patterns.

The various problems caused by coronary artery disease are classified under the general heading of coronary heart disease. Traditionally, people have not become concerned about coronary artery disease until heart problems have arisen. But the epidemic nature of coronary heart disease has forced physicians and the public today to be concerned about the cause as well as its effects.

5

The Three Main Effects
of Coronary Artery Disease

There are three main ways in which hardening of the coronary arteries may show up in the individual:

- with no illness or symptoms,

- with *angina pectoris* ("painful chest"), more commonly known as *angina,*

- with heart attacks (two basic types).

There are two basic types of heart attacks: (1) those causing sudden death, and (2) those known as *acute myocardial infarction.* The latter type is characterized by death of some heart muscle which leads to illness, often of an extended nature, from which recovery is common.

The unpredictable nature of arteriosclerosis is such that the individual with this disease may experience only one of the effects, or he may experience combinations of them in different orders of sequence. For that matter, the effects may in themselves be unpredictable in their course. For example, two individuals harboring similar degrees of coronary arteriosclerosis may have different futures. One may die suddenly without known earlier trouble, while the other may live a full life without any recognizable heart problems. The majority of people with significant coronary arteriosclerosis experience an array of problems lying between these two extremes.

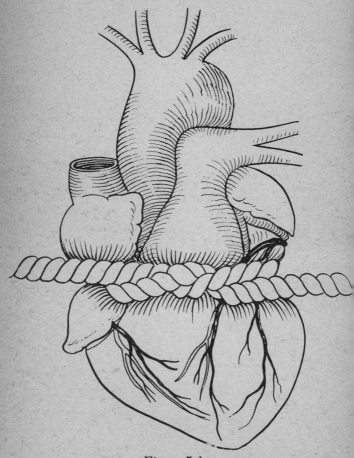

Figure 5-1.

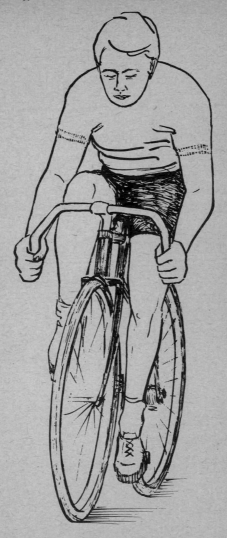

Figure 5-2.

A distinct note of optimism with regard to coronary artery disease is justified. Many persons may have hardening of the coronary arteries for many years without being aware of it. Also, the majority of persons experiencing acute myocardial infarction not only recover but return to productive life after the acute illness has passed.

NO SYMPTOMS OR ILLNESS

A person may have hardening of the coronary arteries without experiencing any recognizable effects. His lack of symptoms or illness means that regardless of the state of his coronary arteries, his heart muscle receives adequate amounts of blood for its needs. However, the fact that such a person may have no symptoms up to a given time does not guarantee him immunity from problems in the future.

One explanation for no symptoms or illness accompanying hardening of the coronary arteries is the presence of certain natural adjustments made by the body. Nature tends to overcome obstructions in coronary arteries by enlargement of small existing arterial connections (collaterals) between the diseased coronary artery and other coronary arteries, thereby providing detours around zones of obstruction.

Part A of Figure 5–3 shows an existing connection between coronary arteries under normal conditions. Part B shows in an exaggerated way how such a collateral has enlarged to carry blood into those portions of the coronary artery affected by the obstruction.

The flow of blood through such detours is called collateral circulation. An effective collateral circulation may explain absence (or even disappearance) of heart problems in the presence of severely obstructive atherosclerosis. In some cases, however, nature's response fails to overcome fully the effects of obstruction.

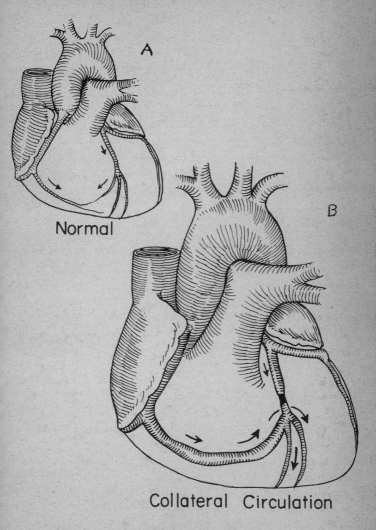

A

B

Normal

Collateral Circulation

Figure 5-3.

Another explanation for the apparent absence of symptoms in a person with hardening of the coronary arteries is that the symptoms have merely gone unnoticed. In other words, minor heart attacks have occurred in his past without his realizing the fact. That is, some of his heart muscle has become damaged or has died from inadequate blood supply (see Chapter 6). The only sign afterward would be a scar in the muscle of the heart. Such unnoticed past heart attacks may or may not show up on an *electrocardiogram* (EKG).

THE ELECTROCARDIOGRAM: NOT A CRYSTAL BALL

The electrocardiogram (see also pages 43 – 45) is a test of the heart muscle, not of the coronary arteries. Therefore, a person with coronary artery disease in whom the heart muscle has not been adversely affected may have a normal EKG. Future muscle damage may result from the arteriosclerosis, but the electrocardiogram is not a crystal ball and cannot predict such effects. It tells only what is going on at the time of the test with regard to the nature and performance of the heart muscle.

There is no easy way to ascertain the presence or precise extent of coronary artery disease in the person who has shown neither symptoms nor electrocardiographic evidence of muscle damage. Everybody should be aware, however, that absence of abnormal electrocardiographic signs does not necessarily mean absence of coronary disease.

ANGINA PECTORIS

Angina pectoris, or more commonly, *angina*, is a term for temporary incidents of chest pain caused by coronary artery disease.

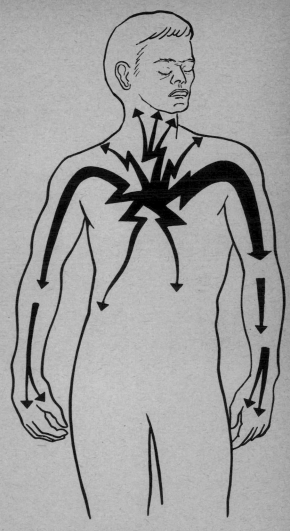

Figure 5-4.

Such incidents of chest pain are common manifestations of coronary arteriosclerosis, and as such provide strong evidence of hardening of the coronary arteries in the affected individual. Those who experience angina have arteriosclerosis which has developed to such an extent that blood flow through the coronary arteries occasionally becomes inadequate for the needs of the heart muscle. Such inadequacy is enough to cause pain (angina) but not enough to cause a heart attack.

Classically, angina is described as an inward pressure or clutching-like pain under the breast bone. It may be mild or severe. This pain may extend to other areas, especially the left arm and less frequently into the right arm, abdomen, neck, or even the teeth. While angina may occur spontaneously when the individual is relaxing, it is usually brought on by physical or emotional exertion and/or by exposure to severe cold. Rest or returning to a warm atmosphere usually relieves the discomfort. Patients for whom nitroglycerin has been prescribed may also find relief by taking this medicine during episodes of angina. Nitroglycerin usually causes the coronary arteries to dilate. When they dilate, the arteries allow more blood to flow to the heart muscle and so relieve the temporary episode.

Other conditions causing chest pains may be confused with angina. These include pleurisy, pericarditis (inflammation over the heart), arthritis of the neck and back, certain diseases of the nerves or of the esophagus, gall stones, diaphragmatic hernia, and others. It is therefore important to realize that some types of chest pain are unrelated to coronary artery disease and therefore not as serious as angina.

The stress exercise or Master's test, an electrocardiogram test taken while the patient exercises, may be used by the physician to determine whether chest pain experienced by a given individual is, in fact, caused by coronary artery disease.

The presence of hardening of the coronary arteries which underlies angina does in some individuals lead to more serious consequences, taking the form of heart attack. If heart attack strikes people with angina, the heart attack may come soon after angina is first recognized, or as happens more often, years later.

But the person with angina need not be pessimistic. Millions of people with angina have not suffered any condition more serious and have continued to be fully productive. Many have even gone through major surgical operations for other diseases without difficulty.

For that matter, the person who experiences the pain of angina may be better off than someone without this symptom who has the same degree of coronary artery disease. The angina is an early warning signal that can help in determining how much exertion can be endured without overtaxing the heart. A person can take advantage of this signal by using greater care in the choice of his activities. By using the onset of angina as a guide concerning degree of work, the affected individual may thus avoid the future onset of angina and, in some instances at least, the precipitation of heart attack.

6

Heart Attack

Heart attack, of which there are two basic types, is the third possible effect of coronary artery disease.

Heart attack is caused by an inadequate supply of blood for the needs of heart muscle and is a more serious response to the deficiency than angina.

Oxygen Bankruptcy

Heart attacks may be understood in terms of *oxygen bankruptcy*. Individuals go financially bankrupt if either of two conditions is present: (1) they have no income or (2) they spend more money than they receive. The same principles apply to heart muscle. If heart muscle (1) receives no blood or (2) uses more oxygen than it receives, it can achieve a state of oxygen bankruptcy. When heart muscle is in this condition, it can bring on either of the two basic types of heart attack.

The two types of heart attack are easily distinguished by the fact that one relates to major disturbance in the heart's signal system, which usually results in sudden death. In the other type, called *acute myocardial infarction*, the basic disturbance is death of heart muscle, which may cause sudden death but usually allows the person enough time to seek medical attention and to become hospitalized. Recovery is the usual outcome.

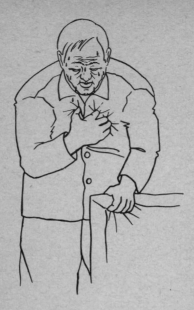

Figure 6-1.

HEART ATTACKS CAUSING SUDDEN DEATH

Heart attacks causing sudden death are the largest single cause of death in the United States. Such heart attacks take the lives of about 250,000 Americans each year, a toll approximating five times the incidence of highway deaths.

The usual basis for heart attacks of the sudden-death variety is disturbance of the electrical system of the heart, which normally coordinates the activities of the individual muscle fibers. That is, the inadequacy of blood flowing through the diseased coronary arteries causes abnormal irritability of heart muscle and complications which lead to so-called electrical failure.

In such failure, each heart muscle fiber beats on its own without waiting for a central signal. The lack of coordination of contraction of the many muscle fibers makes the ventricles ineffective as pumps in a manner reminiscent of the earlier drawing (Figure 2-4) of men unsuccessfully trying to lift a car. The heart merely twitches chaotically and the circulatory system stalls from the lack of a driving force. Such a condition in the heart is known as *ventricular fibrillation*. Its occurrence means that death will follow within a few minutes if proper contraction of the ventricles is not restored.

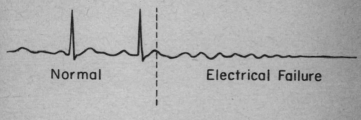

Normal   Electrical Failure

Figure 6-2.

Reference to heart attacks causing "sudden" death may be somewhat misleading, for in many cases the onset of such attacks apparently was preceded by heart muscle damage or warning signs. Autopsies have shown that people dying suddenly from heart attack usually have heart muscle scars, evidencing previous attacks of acute myocardial infarction. Indeed, the scar may have been a factor in initiating the electrical failure.

Certain factors can be helpful in anticipating and averting sudden-death heart attacks. Many people listed as dying suddenly had abnormalities in the day or two before they died. These abnormalities often were symptoms of impending heart attack but were ignored as such. In some instances, the symptoms suggested a problem with another organ, such as the stomach, when in fact they related to a heart problem.

It is advisable for any person with known coronary artery disease to be aware of symptoms of impending heart attack and to report on their appearance to his physician. Among these symptons are:

- persistent angina despite rest or taking of nitroglycerin,

- abnormal degrees of fatigue,

- sweating for no apparent reason,

- the onset of angina at a lower level of work or emotional exertion than was previously required,

- "indigestion."

If the patient is aware of the above symptoms, he can alert his doctor to suspicious signs. His doctor can then evaluate them and provide for appropriate observation and treatment to prevent such consequences as ventricular fibrillation.

When Calvin Coolidge died suddenly in 1933 at the age of sixty, while preparing to shave in his home, the nation was shocked. He had been in excellent health since turning the presidency over to Herbert Hoover in March 1929. In an article on the events leading up to his sudden death, the Associated Press reported: "Mr. Coolidge, following his daily custom, had gone to the office at 8:30 a.m. Seemingly he was in his usual good health. He had complained at times for the past two or three weeks of indigestion but he did not appear to regard his indisposition seriously." Today we believe his death was most likely caused by a sudden-death heart attack involving electrical failure, one early warning of which had been the "indigestion."

Incidentally, not all heart attacks involving major electrical failure spell death. Death occurs only if the condition of ventricular fibrillation goes unchallenged. Given an appropriate amount of time, modern techniques and facilities have the capability of preventing ventricular fibrillation and of overcoming electrical failure. These techniques may prevent sudden death.

Many persons who have died suddenly as the result of major electrical failure have had hearts described as "too good to die." That is, the heart muscle was, for the most part, in good condition. Had the electrical disturbance been corrected, these people might have continued to live for many years. Whenever ventricular fibrillation is overcome, the patient is not necessarily left with a damaged heart or with death of heart muscle. There may be no lingering illness or, for that matter, no further incidents of electrical failure.

ACUTE MYOCARDIAL INFARCTION

Acute myocardial infarction is that type of heart attack in which there is loss of part of the muscle in the left ventricle. Usually the patient survives, but he is left with varying degrees of heart impairment which may or may not cause further problems. Well over one million Americans experience this affliction each year.

Figure 6-3 shows a typical example of acute myocardial infarction. Part of the heart muscle in the left ventricle has been lost (shaded area) and has therefore become ineffective. If the patient survives acute myocardial infarction, the dead muscle in the heart is replaced by a scar. Life then depends upon the ability of the muscle which has survived the attack to pump the blood through the body.

Acute myocardial infarction may occur in an individual without his awareness or concern, as mentioned previously. Such episodes involving the absence of symptoms or the existence of seemingly only minor ones have been called *silent infarction*.

In the more obvious cases, acute myocardial infarction makes itself known to the afflicted in the following ways:

- persistent chest pain or discomfort like angina, despite rest and/or the taking of nitroglycerin (the chest pain may subside temporarily),

- fear of impending death,

- profuse sweating,

- nausea (and vomiting).

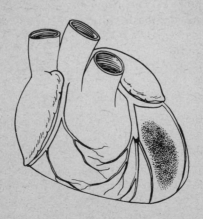

Figure 6-3.

This last sympton has been responsible for the fact that in the past, acute myocardial infarction was at times diagnosed as acute indigestion. President Harding died suddenly in 1923 at the age of fifty-seven while convalescing from an illness considered to be a stomach upset. The official announcement by five doctors who had been caring for Harding said, "The President died instantaneously and without warning and while conversing with members of his family at 7:30 p.m. During the day he had been free from discomfort and there was every justification for anticipating a prompt recovery." His illness characterized acute myocardial infarction which led to sudden death by electrical failure. "Then, all at once, he just went like that," the attending doctor was quoted by the Associated Press. "Just like that; something snapped; that's all."

It is noteworthy that the symptoms of acute myocardial infarction resemble those which may signal an electrical failure and sudden death.

The early effects of an acute myocardial infarction may be mild or severe. The two most serious complications deserve special emphasis. These are (1) electrical failure coming on days or weeks after the death of heart muscle and (2) "pump failure."

ELECTRICAL FAILURE

Arrhythmias (see page 13) of all types may be associated with acute myocardial infarction. But the most serious is electrical failure, the same condition involving uncoordinated contractions which is the usual basis for the heart attack characterized by sudden death. This means that the person with a recent acute myocardial infarction may die suddenly from ventricular fibrillation of the muscle which has survived.

PUMP FAILURE

The other serious complication of acute myocardial infarction is "pump failure." Pump failure means that the left ventricle is ineffective as a pump because of loss of heart muscle. This loss may be the result of one attack of acute myocardial infarction, or the cumulative effects of one attack together with losses of heart muscle from previous attacks. There just isn't enough muscle left to do the job, even with coordinated contractions.

Pump failure and electrical failure represent not only the two most serious potential problems of acute myocardial infarction, but also extremes between which are various types of problems and degrees of illness. Unfortunate, certainly, is the statistical indication that the chances of heart attack are higher for an individual who has already experienced an acute myocardial infarction than for one who has not. On the other hand, thousands of people who have recovered from heart attacks have experienced no further heart problems and have been productive, often returning to their original jobs.

SUSPECT YOUR OWN HEART ATTACK

Many heart attacks cause pain which is unrelenting, severe, and frightening. Individuals experiencing such pain usually suspect a heart attack, and need no coaxing to seek medical attention. Such situations represent no problem to doctors in establishing a diagnosis and instituting appropriate treatment.

Troublesome, however, are heart attacks with less dramatic and less obvious symptoms. Because these attacks are more difficult to sense and to diagnose, they may occur without being reported or attended to. Or a risky period of time may pass before something is done.

It should be emphasized that the consequences of these attacks may be just as serious as those of more obvious attacks. Symptoms do not necessarily indicate the quality or potential of a heart attack. The person with vague symptoms may be unaware of his heart attack and, more important, its potentially serious and even lethal consequences. The longer he waits, the less chance there is for preventing such possible consequences.

Any heart attack may trigger the serious complication of electrical failure, with its high risk of sudden death. Doctors have a better chance of being successful in preventing or overcoming electrical failure in people with acute heart attacks when the patients reach them in time. Obviously, if a heart attack takes place without medical attention, the potentially avoidable sudden death may occur.

As pointed out previously, recent inquiry into cases of sudden death has shown that the death was not infrequently preceded by some illness which caused no particular alarm. But minor abnormalities such as stomach and other disorders may in reality be the symptoms of existing heart attacks or the subtle signs of impending ones.

Again, these seemingly minor symptoms representing the "preamble to death" include excessive fatigue and unexplainable acute attacks of nausea and/or sweating without apparent reason. The persistence of angina despite the employment of measures usually successful in overcoming the pain is also a warning that more serious troubles may lie ahead.

These symptoms are only a few of the manifestations of an existing or impending heart attack. The reader will appreciate, too, that these symptoms may be caused by benign conditions not associated with the heart.

But, since the stakes are high, it seems prudent for the patient and the physician to be sharply attentive to, and extremely concerned about, symptoms of seemingly minor significance—as well as to those of obviously major significance. Stated in another way, it seems preferable for patients and doctors to be overconcerned about minor symptoms than to be underconcerned about major symptoms.

The patient referred to is the individual with known or suspected coronary artery disease and especially anybody who has experienced a heart attack.

Teamwork between the patient and his doctor in a well-balanced program involving the reporting and review of minor symptoms offers the most hopeful and practical means at this time for reducing the high rate of mortality by heart attack. Evaluation of concerned patients who report suspicious symptoms in these uncertain situations will require that medical institutions further develop the capability of short-term (24- to 48-hour) admission of patients for intensive cardiac observation. Employment of such facilities will aid the physician in reassuring the patient who has no cause for concern and in applying timely and appropriate care to the patient who does have cause.

CONFIRMING THE EXISTENCE OF A HEART ATTACK

Because heart attacks are sometimes difficult to recognize and may even go unnoticed by the affected individual, one may wonder how to know for sure that a heart attack is occurring or has occurred. One may also wonder if the extent of muscle damage can be determined.

The diagnosis of a heart attack and the extent of its damage is the responsibility of the physician. His most useful tool in this regard is what the patient reports to him about the symptoms and the details of the suspected heart attack.

The *electrocardiograph* can also be extremely helpful in diagnosing a heart attack if certain abnormalities are present. This is the instrument designed to measure the electrical performance of heart muscle (Figure 6-4).

The electrocardiograph employs sensing devices which are placed on various locations of the body, as shown in the drawing. These devices monitor the electric current present in contractions of heart muscle. The various sensing devices feed into an instrument which prints out patterns on graph paper. This record of printed patterns is called an *electrocardiogram*, or an EKG (see page 28). The physician interprets the patterns, and in this manner may determine the presence, extent, and location of muscle damage in the heart.

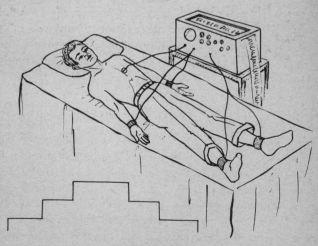

Figure 6-4.

Nevertheless, despite the common use of the electrocardiogram and its high degree of reliability, it is not a crystal ball. It cannot predict a heart attack or future muscle damage. Further, the EKG may not be able to identify certain types of heart attacks, even when present.

The EKG test is usually performed with the patient lying down, as shown. But the test can also be done while the patient exercises in the so-called stress exercise or Master's test (as noted on page 30 with regard to ascertaining whether chest pain is angina).

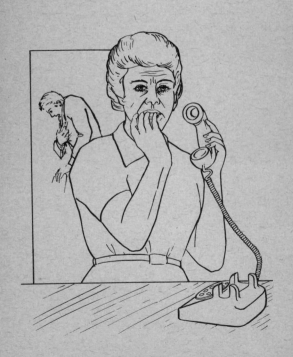

Figure 6-5.

The physician may use other diagnostic procedures to supplement the EKG or to confirm its results. These procedures involve measurement of certain ingredients or qualities of blood on a frequent basis over a period of days. Among the items studied are enzymes, white blood cells, and the so-called sedimentation rate. Their levels rise over normal in acute myocardial infarction. Thus, an increase in the levels from one measurement to the next may help to indicate that some heart muscle has died.

Curiously and importantly, all the tests (including the EKG) may show no evidence of an acute heart attack when the only supporting evidence is the patient's own story. In such circumstances, the patient may well have had a heart attack. Such hard-to-diagnose heart attacks are potentially as dangerous as those which are more obvious.

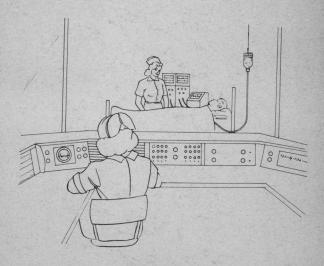

Figure 6-6.

WHEN A HEART ATTACK STRIKES

Most people who suffer acute heart attacks live long enough to receive help if they seek it promptly. The medical profession and other groups stand ready to act fast and to help the heart attack victim through his crisis.

If you suspect a heart attack, don't be embarrassed to call for help: your doctor, the local hospital, the police or fire department. Families should have readily available a list of telephone numbers to call in emergencies such as the occurrence of a heart attack.

The victim of the attack should lie down.

Individuals do not always collapse and lose consciousness during acute heart attacks, but when they do, so-called external cardiac compression and mouth-to-mouth resuscitation are sometimes helpful. However, as a practical matter, the bystanders are usually emotionally upset as well as unacquainted with proper techniques and therefore ineffective in their efforts to help. The interested reader is advised to seek out the first aid courses available in most communities to learn more about assisting the unconscious victim of a heart attack.

If you are the victim, don't be embarrassed to call for help and lie down.

An ambulance or other special vehicle will come to transport the afflicted individual to the hospital, where he will enter the coronary care unit.

THE CORONARY CARE UNIT

The coronary care unit or intensive coronary care unit, as it is sometimes called, receives patients with suspected heart attacks and those in the first few days after the onset of acute myocardial infarction. Its primary purpose is to prevent death due to electrical failure during this critical period. Patients with acute myocardial infarction may experience potentially fatal arrhythmias soon after the onset of the attack.

The coronary care unit is designed:

(1) to monitor heart rhythms with the aid of an electrocardiograph and to make other continuous observations of such indicators of condition as blood pressure, and

(2) to have nurses and other specially trained personnel available for quick treatment of electrical disturbances should these complications appear.

Among the tools of the coronary care unit for the correction of arrhythmias are corrective drugs, pacemakers (to be discussed later), oxygen, and the so-called ventricular defibrillator. This last instrument can restore the contractions in a heart which has gone into the feeble condition of ventricular fibrillation, the usual basis of sudden death.

Other instruments being developed for the coronary care unit are various pump-assistance devices designed to help pump blood throughout the body while the heart is temporarily incapable of doing this job effectively.

The process of recovery from the early, critical days in the coronary care unit is a gradual one. This involves a period in a part of the hospital other than the coronary care unit before returning home.

The patient and his physician must then concern themselves with further and more comprehensive recovery from the heart attack.

7

Recovering from a Heart Attack

A person who has survived acute myocardial infarction is bombarded with concern and advice from his physician, family, and friends. The many comments from a variety of people can cause confusion and even interfere with the full recovery of the patient. The patient has three main objectives for recovery. These are:

(1) overcoming the residual effects of the recent heart attack,

(2) returning to work,

(3) preventing another heart attack.

OVERCOMING THE RESIDUAL EFFECTS

Not all complications from acute myocardial infarction are electrical disturbances. More than half result from muscle or pump failure.

It is important to remember that all patients who have recovered from acute myocardial infarction have had loss of some heart muscle and a scar remains. In the overwhelming number of individuals, the amount of heart muscle lost and, coincidentally, the size of the scar are not so great as to cause major inadequacy of the left ventricle as a pump. But varying degrees of pump inadequacy may linger. Troublesome arrhythmias may also contribute to a heart's inability to do a normal job. For many patients so affected,

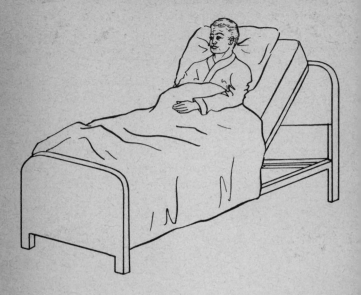

Figure 7-1.

certain forms of surgery may help to remedy the effects if these are not helped effectively by nonsurgical means.

NON-SURGICAL TREATMENT

In most patients who are left with problems, these can be managed by nonsurgical, medical means.

As part of the medical treatment, some physicians include long-term administration of blood thinners (anticoagulants) and, at times, other drugs. Specific treatment for each patient depends upon the doctor's evaluation of the extent of muscle damage, the most critical resulting abnormalities, and the patient's rate of recovery.

Suffice it to say that doctors have available a wide variety of highly effective medical measures which are employed to treat the particular problems of each patient. Most nonsurgical forms of treatment are effective. The vast majority of people who have recovered from acute myocardial infarction do not need surgical treatment for the results of the heart attack.

SURGICAL TREATMENT

If medical management proves to be ineffective, surgical treatment may be recommended, the type of operation depending upon the details in the individual patient.

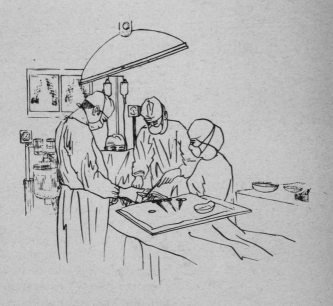

Figure 7-2.

It is important to remember that each of the patients to be operated on has problems in coronary obstruction and therefore is prone to future coronary heart problems. Certain operations have been developed to increase blood flow to heart muscle when such flow has been slowed by coronary obstructions. These patients logically may be candidates for such operations, generally known as *revascularization* procedures.

Such operations are intended to prevent angina and heart attacks. Revascularization surgery is discussed in detail in chapter 8, on heart attack prevention.

In contrast to revascularization procedures, which are primarily intended to prevent angina and heart attack, there are other operations which are designed to overcome certain particular complications of acute myocardial infarction.

Four specific problems resulting from acute myocardial infarction have been treated surgically to help the patient in his recovery. These are abnormalities which are basically mechanical in nature and thus lend themselves to rather immediate correction: arrhythmias, an *aneurysm*, valve insufficiency, and rupture of heart muscle.

With the exception of attaching *pacemakers* to patients for treatment of arrhythmias (see the following section), operations on the heart usually are not performed until one month or longer after the onset of an acute myocardial infarction. The relatively easy and uncomplicated surgery involved with pacemaker devices is the only exception. Pacemakers are sometimes introduced during the acute phase.

The *artificial heart and lung machine*, shown conceptually in Figure 7-3, is one reason for the relatively complicated and planned nature of the so-called open heart operations.

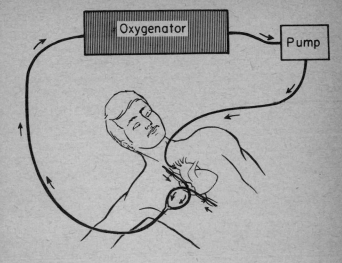

Figure 7-3.

All of the operations to be discussed, except for those related to pacemakers, involve open heart surgery. The surgeon intercepts blood flowing to the heart and directs it through a tube to the heart and lung machine. The machine takes over the oxygenation and pumping of the blood, redirecting the blood back into the patient's circulatory system. Such functions of the heart-lung machine allow the surgeon to stop the patient's heart and work on it. After the operation has been performed, the surgeon restores the normal flow of blood through the heart, and the heart starts beating again while the lungs also come back into function.

ARRHYTHMIAS AND PACEMAKERS

Certain arrhythmias following acute myocardial infarction do not threaten the individual as much as electrical failure. But they may affect the pumping function adversely so that the circulatory system is not completely efficient. Such arrhythmias may lead to electrical failure if not corrected.

Certain medicines usually are effective. In the exceptional case where these are ineffective in correcting such rhythm disturbances, a pacemaker may be employed. Depending on circumstances, a temporary or permanent pacemaker is used. Either is a device with its own batteries adjusted to stimulate the heart electrically at a steady rate. The restoration of a normal rhythm assures adequate frequency and coordination of heart muscle contractions.

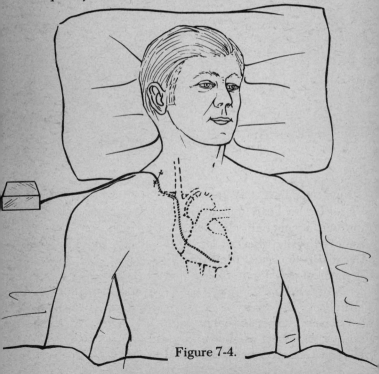

Figure 7-4.

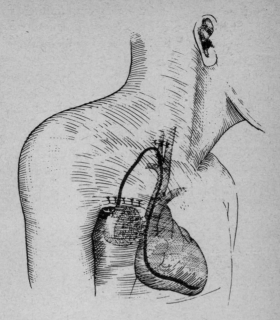

Figure 7-5.

The temporary pacemaker is outside the body. It is connected to heart muscle by way of electrodes passed through a vein into the heart. The electrodes may be removed easily when no longer required. If the patient's status fails to correct itself with a temporary pacemaker, a permanent pacemaker may be used.

The "permanent," or portable, pacemaker is used if the heart lacks the ability to sustain normal rhythms without assistance. The permanent pacemaker is inserted under the skin of the chest as shown in Figure 7-5. From it, the electrical connections extend into the heart through a vein.

Figure 7–6 shows a common type of permanent pacemaker which is about the size of an adult's palm. The batteries may last for two or more years. If the power weakens, the unit may be replaced with another.

The operation for placement or replacement of a pacemaker is a relatively simple one, requiring only local anesthesia, and about one day in the hospital in the usual circumstance. Researchers continue to seek longer-lasting power sources so that replacement of pacemakers will be necessary less often than with current models.

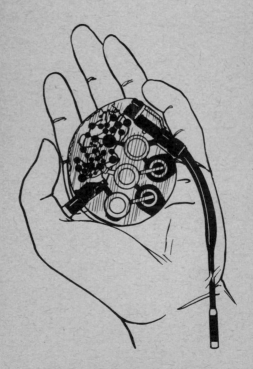

Figure 7-6.

ARRHYTHMIAS AND REMOVAL OF SCAR

Arrhythmias in certain patients may be diagnosed as being caused primarily by the scar, sometimes even a small scar, remaining in the heart muscle after acute myocardial infarction has "healed." In such individuals, if the scar is located in a portion of the left ventricle from which it may be removed without undue hazard, it is, on rare occasions, logical to remove the scar.

Figure 7–7A shows how the surgeon may remove a scar believed to be the main cause of troublesome and otherwise uncontrollable arrhythmias. The removal is followed by a stitching up of the muscle in the main pump, as shown in 7–7B. Irregular heart beats (7–7A) and the resumption of a normal pattern (7–7B) are shown on the electrocardiographic-type representations.

It is to be emphasized that this form of surgical treatment is very unusual for arrhythmias which follow acute myocardial infarction.

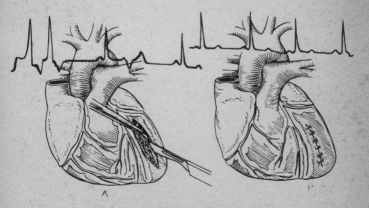

A   B

Figure 7-7.

EXCISION OF A LEFT-VENTRICULAR ANEURYSM

Loss of a large amount of muscle from the left ventricle as a result of an acute myocardial infarction may be associated with a permanent abnormal bulge in the left ventricle. The bulge may develop in the weeks, months, or years following the episode of acute myocardial infarction.

The bulge is called an *aneurysm* (Figure 7–8). It is walled by fibrous tissue and does not contribute to the total contractile force of the main pump. Much worse, it expands outward when the functioning heart muscle contracts, thereby dissipating some important energy that

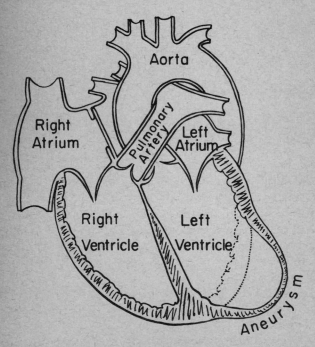

Figure 7-8.

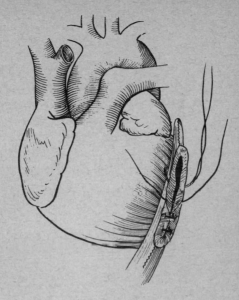

Figure 7-9.

otherwise would go toward the movement of blood forward through the body. This condition may cause *chronic heart failure*, a continuing inability of the main pump to move enough blood to sustain the normal operations of the body. Under such circumstances, it is appropriate to excise the aneurysm so as to make the work of the contracting heart muscle more efficient. The operation is called an *aneurysmectomy*.

After the aneurysm is removed, the remaining muscle is sewn together, leaving a main pump that is near normal in size and shape.

Aneurysmectomy is not suggested for all left-ventricular aneurysms, one reason being that if the scar is very large, its removal would leave a left ventricle too small for normal pumping.

Other aneurysms are poorly situated for surgical removal. For example, an aneurysm may be located where it involves muscle relating to the mitral valve. The mitral valve controls the opening between the left atrium and left ventricle. The valve opens to allow the flow of blood into the left ventricle. Its closure prevents the flow of blood back into the atrium when the ventricle contracts. Removal of an aneurysm so located may upset the function of the mitral valve and leave it unable to close. The result is leakage which reduces the effectiveness of the main pump. In some of these situations the surgeon may attempt to replace the natural mitral valve with an artificial one while also removing the aneurysm. This is a logical though a high-risk procedure.

REPLACEMENT OF THE MITRAL VALVE

Incompetence or leakage of the mitral valve in the absence of an aneurysm is another possible late effect of an acute myocardial infarction. (The function of the mitral valve is described in the previous section: Excision of a Left-Ventricular Aneurysm.) This condition may result from rupture of specialized muscle which supports the mitral valve or, more commonly, from scarring of this muscle. Especially in the latter situation, certain drugs may remedy the problem and so make an operation unnecessary.

In some cases, the affected mitral valve is replaced surgically with an artificial valve. Figure 7–10 shows one common type of artificial valve, the ball valve, after it has been sewn into place.

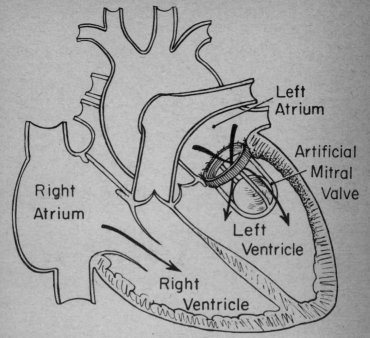

Figure 7-10.

REPAIR OF RUPTURE

Another consequence of acute myocardial infarction may be rupture of the wall (septum) between the main pump (left ventricle) and the auxiliary pump (right ventricle). Fortunately, this complication is uncommon.

The rupture occurs during the early stages of acute myocardial infarction and is dangerous. Some patients survive the immediate effects of the rupture but are ill because of the abnormal flow of blood through the new opening and the resulting strain upon the left ventricle.

The smaller drawing in Figure 7–11 shows such a rupture. Closure of the opening with a patch, as shown in the larger drawing, is the appropriate surgical treatment. If the patient's condition permits, the operation is usually delayed until scar tissue has replaced the dead muscle at the edges of the opening. The reason for the delay is that the presence of scar tissue allows a more secure closure.

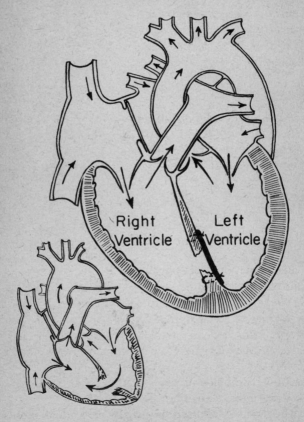

Right Ventricle

Left Ventricle

Figure 7-11.

EXTENSIVE PUMP FAILURE

The foregoing surgical procedures relate to problems contributing to various degrees of ineffectiveness in the pumping of blood by the heart as possible consequences of an acute myocardial infarction.

If there is massive loss of heart muscle, as a result of one or several attacks of acute myocardial infarction, pump failure may be so extensive that the operations described won't help. For such an unfortunate condition, *heart transplantation* has been employed. But heart transplants have led only to questionable or disappointing results.

ARTIFICIAL HEARTS

Experiments are continuing in the development of man-made devices to be used instead of transplanted hearts. These devices, called *artificial hearts* or *artificial ventricles,* are designed to be implanted in the patient. Their main purpose will be to take over the work of the main pump on a permanent basis. At the present time, no such device is available.

RETURN TO WORK

After treatment of specific residual effects, if any, of an acute heart attack, the second objective in the recovery of the patient is his return to work. It is important for the individual to realize that in the majority of instances, people who have recovered from myocardial infarction have returned to their original job or a modification of it. There are many examples of individuals who have continued in office or have assumed major public service positions after recovery.

The course followed is usually a gradual increase in activity commensurate with the heart's effectiveness as a

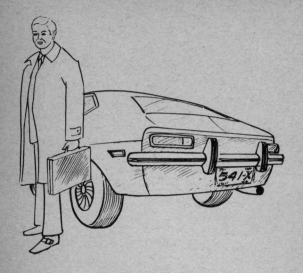

Figure 7-12.

pump and its response to stepped-up demands. This approach allows return to work at varying times depending upon the patient's condition. Return to work may be in the person's usual job or in one less strenuous. Shortness of breath, fatigue, or chest pain suggest to the individual and to his physician that the work is too strenuous and the job assignment should be modified.

Don't Give Up!

Some people recovering from an acute heart attack tend to give up. They may not attempt to return to work at all. If they return to their job and a symptom such as angina appears, they may be so discouraged as to retreat from all work. This attitude is generally most inadvisable. Individuals who give up tend to carry an emotional strain which is potentially more dangerous than some satisfying work.

Physicians are prepared to work with the individual to help assure satisfying reemployment and to place a proper perspective on his physical condition. Other persons who have recovered from myocardial infarction will receive advice and opinions of others who have experienced the same condition. It should be recalled that each person's condition is not exactly like that of another person. Persons who have recovered can often, with good reason, give encouragement by example to the person who is recovering. Medical advice should be reserved for the physician who is familiar with the details of the given patient's case.

PREVENTION OF ANOTHER HEART ATTACK

Prevention of another heart attack is the third objective in the patient's recovery.

One logical approach would seem to be the attempt to clear up the coronary obstructions which caused the original attack and would be the basis of another attack. For example, patients and their families often enter into "crash programs" of diet after the occurrence of a heart attack. They assume that if the diet has had an influence on the development of coronary artery disease, a change in diet can clear up or reverse arteriosclerosis.

This expectation is unrealistic. In the patient who has had a heart attack, hardening of the coronary arteries has developed to such an extent that the condition cannot be reversed or at least to no appreciable degree. Even how much its further development can be completely halted is uncertain.

Diet may help to prevent worsening of the condition. It may also serve to lower the patient's weight, with the beneficial effect of reduced work for the afflicted heart. If the patient has high blood pressure, reduction in weight is one favorable factor in lowering blood pressure. But one cannot expect miracles from diet or any other approaches known today to clear up obstructions in diseased coronary arteries. Such measures can help to prevent worsening of the arteriosclerosis, but can in no way eliminate it.

There is also the direct attempt to avoid another heart attack in the presence of the diseased coronary arteries. Certain measures can help to prevent heart attacks, and thus efforts along these lines are realistic for persons who have had a heart attack.

The approach to prevention for these people, then, is twofold. It employs measures specifically designed to prevent another heart attack and includes efforts to prevent worsening of the coronary arteriosclerosis. A detailed discussion of such preventive approaches follows.

8

Preventive Approaches to Coronary Heart Disease

An intelligent approach to prevention in coronary heart disease requires that one understand what he is trying to prevent.

It has been pointed out that formation of arteriosclerosis may be followed by progression of the disease. Eventually, the diseased coronary arteries may become so obstructed as to cause angina or heart attack. The sequence of formation, progression, and effects of coronary artery disease contains the logical focal points for prevention.

The person without evidence of coronary arteriosclerosis may not be concerned about heart disease but can be encouraged to orient himself to:

(1) prevention of formation of hardening of the coronary arteries, and

(2) prevention of progression of arteriosclerosis if the disease has already formed.

The individual with known hardening of the coronary arteries must be concerned with two things, namely:

(1) prevention of an initial or subsequent heart attack from the coronary arteriosclerosis, and

(2) prevention of progression of the coronary artery disease.

PRIMARY AND SECONDARY PREVENTION

Prevention of the coronary arteries relates to the fundamental cause of heart attacks, and thus is called "primary prevention." Prevention of heart attacks in the presence of ongoing coronary arteriosclerosis is called "secondary prevention."

PRIMARY PREVENTION

Primary prevention, the prevention of formation or progression of coronary artery disease, is the first priority for the concerned individual who has not evidenced arteriosclerosis in such unmistakable ways as angina or a heart attack. If coronary artery disease is not allowed to form or to progress, coronary heart problems are lessened.

The exact steps of primary prevention are not fully established. This is because such prevention relates to a complex of factors which by themselves and especially in combinations lead to hardening of the coronary arteries. Some of these factors may be unknown today. Others are known, but not yet completely understood. Still others are such that individuals may have little or no control over them.

Primary prevention involves an awareness of these factors coupled with an effort by the person and his physician to do something about them whenever possible. They have been called "risk factors" rather than causes because their presence has been associated with a strong tendency to cause coronary arteriosclerosis.

The risk factors identified as having an influence on the development of coronary artery disease will be discussed separately in the following pages. They are:

(1) genetic background,
(2) blood pressure,

(3) levels of fatty substances in the blood and diet,
(4) sedentary living and obesity,
(5) derangements of chemicals in the blood,
(6) cigarette smoking, *
(7) physical and emotional stress. *

SUSPECT YOUR OWN CORONARY DISEASE

These risk factors are not symptoms of coronary artery disease. However, the presence of one or more should indicate to the individual his potential for having arteriosclerosis to some degree. This does not mean that he will necessarily have coronary heart problems. But he should be aware that he is among the group that tends to and for whom, therefore, preventive measures are especially appropriate.

Awareness of the risk factors in this manner stimulates the individual without evidence of coronary arteriosclerosis to pay attention to the matter of primary prevention.

GENETIC BACKGROUND

It is recognized that the development of hardening of the coronary arteries has a close relationship to family history. Indeed, genetic background may be the strongest factor of all in this disease.

Coronary artery disease is more likely to develop in people whose blood relatives have had the disease. On the other hand, absence of family history of arteriosclerosis does not mean immunity from it.

---

*While cigarette smoking and physical and emotional stress may figure strongly in bringing on a heart attack in an individual with hardening of the coronary arteries, some controversy and uncertainty exist as to whether each has a stimulating effect on the underlying arteriosclerosis.

The influence of genetic background shows up dramatically in both the presence and absence of the disease. There are families with a history of arteriosclerosis at early ages, even when other factors contributing to arteriosclerosis are absent. Other families have shown a history of long life and little coronary artery disease in the presence of many factors which favor the development of the disease.

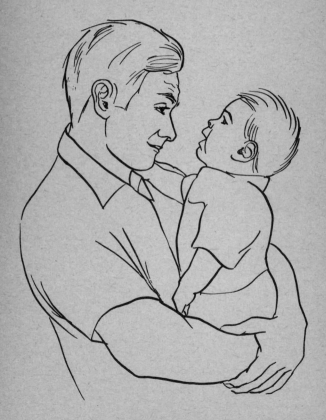

Figure 8-1.

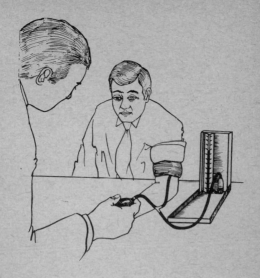

Figure 8-2.

BLOOD PRESSURE

High blood pressure, commonly known as *hypertension*, is associated with the development of hardening of the coronary arteries.

It is fortunate that the medical profession in recent years has had considerable success in lowering the blood pressure of hypertensive patients. This fortunate experience has many health advantages, including the lessening of the tendency for the development or progression of coronary arteriosclerosis. The ease with which blood pressures are taken and the relative ease of correcting hypertension in many individuals make the control of high blood pressure a practical and important step in the prevention of coronary arteriosclerosis.

LEVELS OF FATTY SUBSTANCES IN THE BLOOD AND DIET

Studies of large groups of people have suggested a correlation between coronary heart disease and the level of fatty substances in the blood (often measured as *serum cholesterol*) and diet. Population groups having relatively high levels of serum cholesterol have shown a higher incidence of coronary heart disease than population groups having normal serum cholesterol levels. Within such groups there are exceptions.

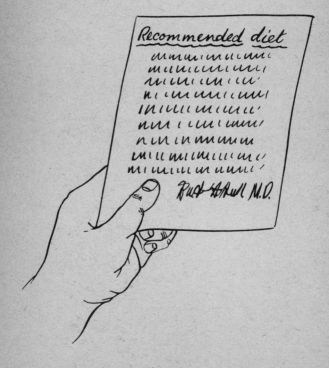

Figure 8-3.

There is a correlation between the dietary intake of animal fats and serum cholesterol levels. This being the case, diet offers a logical approach for the prevention of arteriosclerosis. If pertinent, it presents a realistic challenge for the affluent society to institute a meaningful program of diet for the prevention of coronary artery disease.

The ready availability of rich foods for which we have developed a taste is one stumbling block in such programs. Another very important problem is a tendency to get serious about preventing coronary arteriosclerosis only after it has developed and a heart attack has occurred. In general, relatively little attention is given to this subject by those not yet affected.

For the dietary approach to be successful in the prevention of coronary heart disease, it should apply to the entire family before anyone is afflicted and not restricted to "the man of the house" who has had a heart attack. Logically, it should be started during childhood or at least adolescence. For it is at this time in life that:

(1) the foundation for hardening of the arteries is laid,

and

(2) likes and dislikes for various foods are established.

Difficulties in establishing a well-balanced dietary program stem in part from limited knowledge as to the "good foods" and the "bad foods."

In general, fats derived from animals other than fish are usually "saturated" and have a tendency to cause an elevation in serum cholesterol. Fish fats, liquid oils, and fats of vegetable origin in general are "unsaturated" and do not have this effect. However, liquid vegetable oils which have been made solid (hydrogenated) lose some of their desirable qualities. They become more like the animal fats with a contributory effect on elevating levels of serum cholesterol in the blood.

DIETARY RECOMMENDATIONS

The following dietary recommendations were made by national leaders in the field of arteriosclerosis. These recommendations appeared in a 1970 report of the Inter-Society Commission for Heart Disease Resources, published in *Circulation,* December 1970:

"Americans should be encouraged to modify habits with regard to all five major sources of fat in the U.S. diet—meats, dairy products, baked goods, eggs, table and cooking fats. Specifically a superior pattern of nutrient intake can be achieved by altering habits along the following lines:

"Use lean cuts of beef, lamb, pork, and veal, cooked to dispose of saturated fat and eaten in moderate portion sizes;

"Use lean meat of poultry and fish;

"Use fat-modified (reduced saturated fat and cholesterol content) processed meat products (frankfurters, sausage, salami, etc.);

"Use organ meats (e.g., liver) and shellfish in moderation since they are higher in cholesterol than muscle of red meat, chicken, and fish;

"Avoid fat cuts of meat, addition of saturated fat in cooking meat, large meat portions, and processed meats high in saturated fat;

"Use low-fat and fat-modified dairy products;

"Avoid high-saturated-fat dairy products;

"Use fat-modified baked goods (pies, cookies, cakes, sweet rolls, doughnuts, crullers);

"Avoid baked goods high in saturated fat and cholesterol;

"Use salad and cooking oils, new soft margarines, and shortenings low in saturated fat;

"Avoid butter, margarine, and shortening high in saturated fat;

"Avoid egg yolk, bacon, lard, suet;

"Avoid candies high in saturated fat;

"Use grains, fruits, vegetables, legumes."

FAMILIAL HYPERLIPIDEMIA

A relationship between diet and the level of fatty substances (lipids) in the blood may be demonstrated in most people. There are, however, some individuals with an overwhelming amount of fatty substances in the blood seemingly unrelated to dietary intake of fats. These excessive amounts may be as much as ten times what is considered an abnormally high level.

There is unfortunately in such individuals a strong family tendency for uncontrollable development and progression of arteriosclerosis. The family tendency is recognized in the techical name for the condition: *familial hyperlipidemia*. Individuals in families with this condition may suffer heart attacks as children. While dietary attempts to alter the level of fats in the blood have some effect, they are unfortunately of minor impact in such persons.

Sedentary Living and Obesity

Studies have shown a higher incidence of coronary artery disease among inactive people than among those who are active and exercise regularly. People leading sedentary lives are often obese and thus a relationship between arteriosclerosis and obesity has been suggested as well.

Exercise programs provide a popular means for people to become active and to improve their physical well-being. Whereas exercise may have many beneficial effects, physicians disagree as to its effectiveness in the specific matter of preventing arteriosclerosis. There is no concrete evidence that exercise will prevent coronary artery disease or slow the progression of it once present.

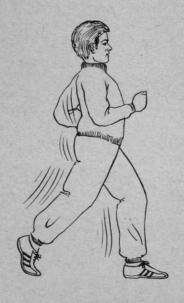

Figure 8-4.

Those who see merit in exercise point out that a prudent, well-supervised program leads to a sense of well-being, to weight control with a related favorable effect on blood pressure, and to a possible stimulus for the development of collateral circulation around obstructed zones in the coronary arteries. Others warn that if exercise exceeds certain critical levels, it can create serious risks for the person with coronary artery disease.

It is generally recommended that adults see their doctor and have a physical examination before entering into an exercise program. The level of activity should be prescribed by the physician. It should begin modestly and build gradually. People with known coronary artery disease should avoid competitive exercise. Those who have had heart attacks and are exercising during rehabilitation should use special caution. With many such people the activity of walking may be sufficient.

OBESITY

Despite the fact that obesity is present in many individuals who suffer coronary heart problems, there is no proof that the condition causes hardening of the coronary arteries. Those who attempt to prevent obesity or lose weight help to prevent arteriosclerosis indirectly. They usually reduce blood pressure as they lose weight. Their diets tend to lower the level of fatty substances in the blood. For these reasons, the prevention of obesity applies to primary prevention.

DERANGEMENTS OF CHEMICALS IN THE BLOOD

Various substances (hormones) are delivered into the circulating blood by certain organs such as the sex organs, the pancreas, and the thyroid gland. Most of these hormones tend to restrain the development of arteriosclerosis. When they are deficient, the restraint is lost and arteriosclerosis tends to develop earlier and more severely than in persons in whom these hormones are more abundant.

Sex hormones are believed to be the reason for the difference in the tendencies of males and females to develop arteriosclerosis during the childbearing years of life. There is a greater incidence of coronary heart disease in men during these years. Women have a much greater incidence of coronary heart disease after the menopause than before. In general, the average age of women with heart attacks is ten years older than that of men. Women from whom the ovaries have been removed during the childbearing years have a tendency to develop coronary arteriosclerosis at a younger age than women with normal ovarian function.

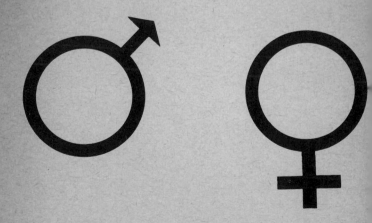

Figure 8-5.

Diabetes, the very common condition which results from inadequate secretion of the hormone insulin by the pancreas, has a stimulating effect on the development of hardening of the coronary arteries. The control of diabetes through diet and use of various medications may possibly have the added benefit of helping the diabetic in primary prevention.

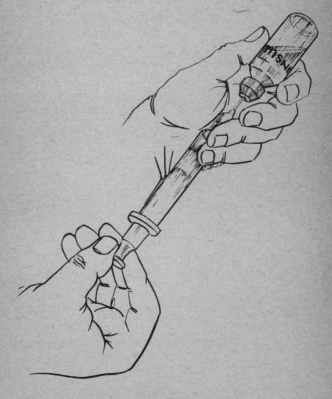

Figure 8-6.

HYPOTHYROIDISM

The thyroid gland, which is situated in the neck, secretes a hormone called thyroxin. This substance has an important controlling influence on metabolism in the various tissues of the body. In certain diseases of the thyroid gland, there is overproduction of thyroxin, leading to a clinical condition known as *hyperthyroidism*.

In other individuals with thyroid disease the reverse is true. Underproduction of thyroxin characterizes a condition called *hypothyroidism* or *myxedema*. This condition has a stimulating effect on the development of arteriosclerosis. This stimulating influence may be corrected by the appropriate medical treatment which overcomes the hypothyroidism or myxedema.

GOUT

Gout is an internal chemical derangement in the body's handling of proteins. Its principal manifestation is pain or swelling of the joints in the extremities. The kidneys may also be affected.

Patients with gout are recognized as having a greater tendency for arteriosclerosis than occurs on the average. Special diets and medicine help to control gout. The control of gout in turn may possibly help to lessen the tendency for arteriosclerosis which accompanies this condition.

CIGARETTE SMOKING

Considerable publicity has been given to the harmful effects of cigarette smoking. With regard to coronary heart disease, there is strong evidence of an association between cigarette smoking and precipitation of heart attack in individuals with hardening of the coronary arteries. As to the relationship between cigarette smoking and development of coronary arteriosclerosis, there is still uncertainty.

PHYSICAL AND EMOTIONAL STRESS

Physical and emotional stress have not been established as factors causing arteriosclerosis. As with cigarette smoking, these factors have evidenced a greater influence on the precipitation of heart attacks in individuals who have hardening of the coronary arteries than on the development of the underlying arteriosclerosis.

SECONDARY PREVENTION

Secondary prevention, the preventive approach aimed directly at avoiding heart attack, is the foremost concern of the individual known to have hardening of the coronary arteries. Since many people may have arteriosclerosis without evidence of it, secondary prevention applies not only to those with known coronary disease but to adults in general.

CONFIRMING THE PRESENCE OF ARTERIOSCLEROSIS

The presence of coronary arteriosclerosis may be assumed when any of the following four abnormalities is identified. It should also be noted that individuals may have none of these and still have coronary arteriosclerosis:

(1) presence of angina pectoris,

(2) history of heart attack from which the individual has recovered,

(3) certain abnormal electrocardiographic signs,

(4) abnormal coronary arteriograms.

CORONARY ARTERIOGRAPHY

Coronary arteriography is a fairly recently developed diagnostic procedure which allows the physician to see the location and extent of obstructions in coronary arteries. It is the only method available today for direct identification of coronary arteriosclerosis. This procedure, also known as *angiography*, uses X-ray techniques and involves inserting a tube called a catheter into the groin or arm. From this point, the catheter is advanced through the aorta to a level just above the heart. The catheter is then directed into the two main coronary arteries, one at a time.

When the catheter is in a coronary artery, dye is injected into the artery. The flow of the dyed blood shows up on X-rays as the blood moves through the coronary artery and its various branches.

Obstructed areas appear on the filmed recordings, which are called *arteriograms*. Arteriograms of left coronary arteries are shown in Figure 8–7.

Because of the relatively complicated nature of this diagnostic procedure, it is performed in special cases. The exact identification of the state of the coronary arteries by

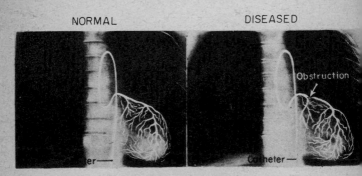

Figure 8-7.

this method forms an important basis in advising one form of treatment or another. The test also helps to determine, in the face of otherwise equivocal evidence, whether or not coronary arteriosclerosis is present.

Whatever the means by which hardening of the coronary arteries is identified, individuals having this condition today are the candidates for heart attacks tomorrow.

The following measures of secondary prevention help to reduce the chances of a heart attack for such people. They will be discussed separately in the following pages. They are:

(1) a well-balanced program of work, rest, and emotional ease,

(2) control of weight,

(3) avoidance of cigarette smoking,

(4) use of primary prevention to halt further progression of coronary arteriosclerosis,

(5) revascularization surgery (for overcoming arterial obstructions which may be particularly severe and threatening).

A WELL-BALANCED PROGRAM OF WORK, REST, AND EMOTIONAL EASE

This ideally includes recreational or work exercise at levels under that which brings on angina or unusual fatigue. Too much rest could represent an imbalance. Some activity is desirable if it is not overdone.

Because emotional stress may play an important role along with physical stress in the precipitation of a heart attack, the program should avoid, if possible, buildup of emotional pressure but provide for proper amounts of physical activity and rest.

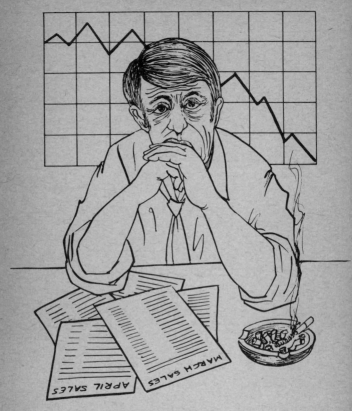

Figure 8-8.

CONTROL OF WEIGHT

The heart with coronary artery disease has a limited capacity for expenditure of energy and performance of work. Obesity compounds the problem by placing a burden of its own on the heart. If coronary artery disease is present, the limited blood flowing through the diseased arteries may not be able to keep up with the increased need for oxygen and nourishment by the working heart muscle. Heart attack may result.

The overweight person commits his heart to a wasteful expenditure of energy and work simply by carrying around the excess weight. Because control of weight reduces the work load on the heart, it improves the capacity of the diseased heart for performance of work and in so doing, lessens the chances of heart attack.

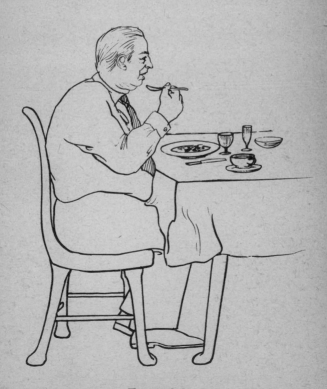

Figure 8-9.

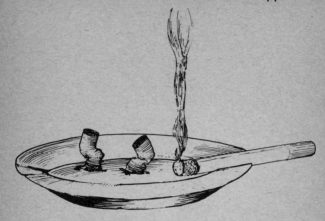

Figure 8-10.

AVOIDANCE OF CIGARETTE SMOKING

Studies relating cigarette smoking to heart attack have shown a direct relationship between the number of cigarettes smoked per day and the tendency to have heart attack.

Without regard to other effects of cigarette smoking, it makes good sense for the individual with potential for a heart attack to avoid cigarettes or at least excessive smoking of them.

USES OF PRIMARY PREVENTION TO HALT FURTHER PROGRESSION OF ARTERIOSCLEROSIS

The foregoing measures aimed specifically at prevention of heart attack for individuals with arteriosclerosis may be supplemented by aspects of primary prevention. Restraining progression of arteriosclerosis will help to lessen the chances of heart attack.

It has been pointed out that there are no means available for the elimination of obstructive deposits in the coronary arteries once they have developed. But primary prevention can be helpful in slowing or halting the further progression of the arteriosclerosis.

All aspects of primary prevention are applicable. Therefore, the person concerned with secondary prevention should know them and use them.

It will be recalled that among the various aspects of primary prevention are employment of measures to control such conditions as high blood pressure, diabetes, hypothyroidism, and gout. Also recommended is attention to diet in an effort to lower the intake of fatty substances. The interested reader is advised to review the preceding section on primary prevention (pages 68 – 81).

REVASCULARIZATION SURGERY

When the coronary arteries are so diseased as to cause overriding concern for the supply of blood to heart muscle, the physician can turn to revascularization surgery. In selected patients this aspect of secondary prevention may be an immediate and potentially effective way to prevent heart attacks.

Revascularization surgery aims to improve the supply of blood to heart muscle. As such, it represents one of the most dramatic breakthroughs of recent years in the treatment of coronary heart disease. For the first time, man has been able surgically to improve the delivery of blood to heart muscle in individuals with coronary arteriosclerosis.

Several revascularization surgical procedures have been developed over the past ten years. Refinements and new ideas continue to appear, and it seems certain that the future will bring new as well as improved techniques.

These operations are performed on individuals with highly developed coronary artery disease. Such individuals have most often been the recent victims of myocardial infarction. Those with severe problems have an obvious need and usually warrant surgery more urgently than people with coronary artery disease who have not had heart attacks. The surgery in such cases has rehabilitative effects while it also helps to prevent another attack.

For the person with threatening degrees of coronary artery disease who has not experienced acute myocardial infarction, the surgery may help to prevent an initial heart attack by improving the supply of blood to the heart muscle. The decision to operate should properly be made by a team consisting of the patient's physician, a cardiologist, and a surgeon.

Prior to any revascularization operation, the physician studies the patient's coronary arteries with coronary arteriography. The special X-ray diagnosis shows the extent and locations of the obstructions in the diseased arteries, as explained earlier in this chapter (page 82). The function of the left ventricle is also studied. With this information, the medical team can decide on the desirability of revascularization surgery, the type of operation if one is warranted, and the surgeon's strategy for overcoming the particular distribution of obstructions in the patient.

THE VINEBERG PROCEDURE

One of the earliest procedures employed was the so-called *Vineberg procedure*, introduced by Dr. Arthur Vineberg of Montreal. In this procedure, which under certain circumstances continues in use today, the surgeon makes use of one of the *internal mammary arteries*. These arteries lie under the breastbone and normally do not run

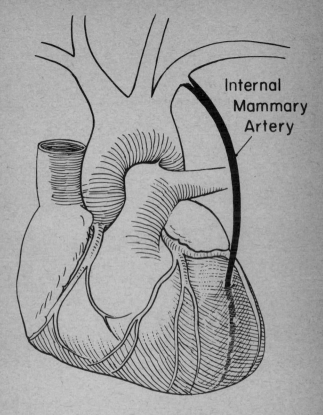

Internal
Mammary
Artery

Figure 8-11.

to the heart. The surgeon implants the end of one artery into the heart muscle but not directly into a coronary artery. The theory and apparent fact is that heart muscle can absorb and use some of the blood which flows from this new source. In this operation, the coronary arteries are not directly operated upon.

Revascularization surgical procedures which were developed after the Vineberg operation work directly on the diseased coronary arteries.

REMOVAL OF DEPOSITS

One of the surgical procedures involving the coronary arteries directly is the so-called *coronary endarterectomy*. Carbon dioxide gas is injected into the wall of the artery so as to loosen the abnormal deposits. The surgeon then makes an incision and removes the obstructive material. The intended result is that the "cleaning out" of the artery will allow blood to flow more freely into the heart muscle.

The operation's concept is logical. However, the endarterectomy is performed only occasionally. One reason that it is not widely used is that severely diseased arteries usually have numerous obstructions and removal of one or even more may have only a minor effect on the flow of blood. There is also the chance of clotting on the raw surfaces left after the deposits have been removed.

SURGICALLY CREATED DETOURS AROUND OBSTRUCTIONS

The most widely used of the current procedures also involves work done directly on the coronary arteries. But rather than attempting to remove the obstructive deposits, the surgeon creates "detours" around them. He borrows veins or arteries from other parts of the body and makes them into alternate routes. These alternate routes are detours through which blood can flow from the aorta into coronary arteries beyond obstructed areas.

The procedure has attracted much publicity and acclaim because it is the most recent, most widely used, and most successful of the various revascularization procedures. It is called *aorto-coronary artery bypass grafting*.

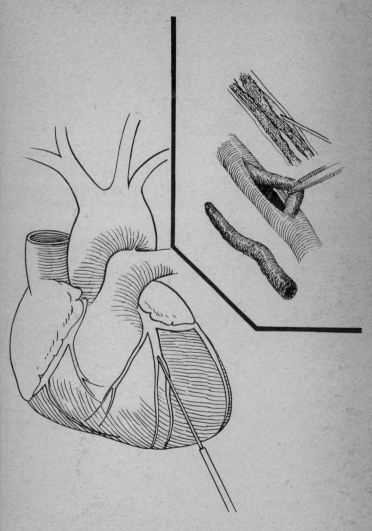

Figure 8-12.

Vein Graft

One version of the bypass procedure involves the use of a borrowed vein. It is known simply as the *vein bypass* or *vein graft* operation. The surgeon removes a vein from the leg of the patient. One end of the vein is connected to the aorta, the other to the coronary artery at a point beyond the obstructed area, as shown in Figure 8–13.

In this manner, the effects of the obstructions are overcome. The vein graft brings an increased amount of blood to the coronary artery beyond the obstructed area. The same pressure which causes the blood to flow through the bypass forces the blood to continue through the coronary artery. The lower portion of the diseased coronary artery is thus enabled to continue its normal function of distributing blood to heart muscle.

The drawing shows only one vein graft connected to the right coronary artery. Depending on the condition in the diseased heart, two or more vein bypasses may be constructed by the surgeon to carry blood to either or both coronary arteries.

Arterial Bypass

The other version of the bypass operation involves the use of one or two borrowed arteries rather than veins. It is called the *arterial bypass* or *arterial graft* operation.

The two arteries are those which are also used in the Vineberg procedure (see page 88). These are the two internal mammary arteries which originate from the aorta and extend to either side of the breastbone.

Figure 8–14 shows both of these arteries after they have been freed up and directed to the heart. In the Vineberg procedure, the internal mammary artery is carried to heart muscle, whereas in the arterial graft operation the artery is

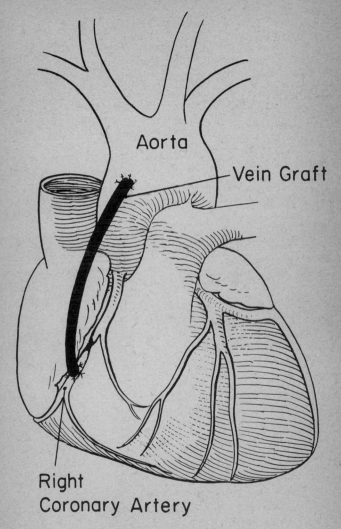

Figure 8-13.

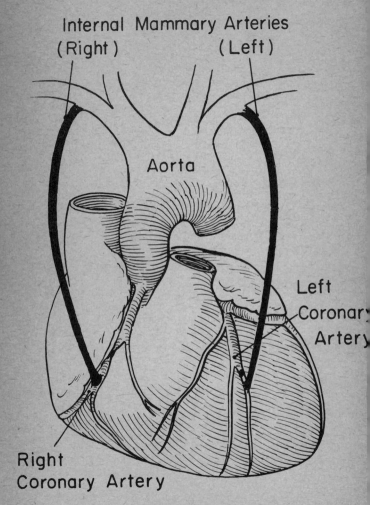

Figure 8-14.

carried into a coronary artery. The lower end is connected to the coronary artery beyond the obstructed area. The intended result of the arterial bypass is the same as in the vein graft operation.

Whether a vein or artery is used for the bypass depends on several factors, such as the locations of the obstructions in the coronary arteries, the number of grafts needed, and the size of the patient's internal mammary arteries.

Revascularization surgery is a profoundly important new means of treating obstructive coronary atherosclerosis and possibly of preventing heart attacks. It has significant prospects for the future as well.

But within the total context of prevention, it should be viewed in proper perspective. Ideally, the preventive approach begins early in life with a view toward prevention of the formation of coronary artery disease. The focus on primary prevention continues with benefits toward the prevention of progression of the disease.

The person who succeeds in this manner assures himself of the special privilege of considering revascularization surgery as a matter of interest and not one of personal necessity.

9

The Future

The future in the field of coronary heart disease and heart attack presents a number of hurdles. Some of these hurdles may be overcome by greater public awareness of the problems in combination with an ever-increasing investigation by the medical profession.

In the area of prevention, the control of high blood pressure, diabetes, hypothyroidism, and gout offers tangible preventive approaches when there is close cooperation between the afflicted and his physician.

The dietary approach to prevention of arteriosclerosis has many challenges. It requires knowledge of the diets best suited to prevent the disease and willingness of all family members, including children, to follow such diets. The food industry can contribute by making readily available those foods which tend to prevent abnormally high accumulations of fatty substances in the blood.

For the person with coronary arteriosclerosis, there may be better methods for preventing heart attacks than at present. A major step in the right direction may come from a greater awareness by the public of the early signs of heart attack. This, coupled with the physician's use of coronary care units as a facility for early observation of the patient, may very well save more people from sudden death.

For the person experiencing a heart attack, greater use of coronary care units and postcoronary care observation in the hospital are attractive means of preventing serious and even fatal complications. In this connection, further development of methods should be forthcoming to assist the circulation during the trying days of severe pump failure which may accompany acute myocardial infarction.

Meanwhile, pharmaceutical researchers and the medical profession are working to improve drugs and methods for treating organs other than the heart which may also be affected by a heart attack.

Surgery for coronary artery disease has currently entered into the exciting stage wherein obstructed segments of the coronary arteries are bypassed by grafts. As in any field, time and experience are certain to improve techniques of this new procedure.

The difficult problem of treating the patient with extensive loss of heart muscle and consequent pump failure is yet to be solved. Heart transplantation has not given the generally favorable results which were envisioned at the time the operation first appeared.

This leaves for the ingenuity of man the development of devices, the so-called artificial hearts, which someday may prove to be the only lifesaving measure in the patient who cannot benefit from any other means.

As Dr. Paul Dudley White points out in the Foreword, we do not have all the answers but we now know enough to do something about coronary heart disease. Indeed, "we have got to roll up our sleeves and work at it."

Index

HEALTH and MEDICINE BOOKS